The Anti-Aging Diet

Discover The Foods That Fight Aging

RON KNESS

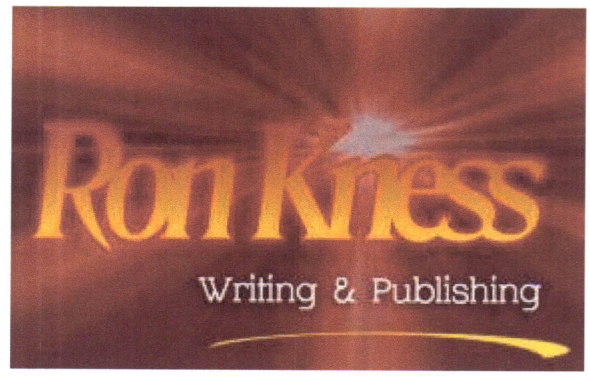

Copyright © 2017 Ron Kness

All rights reserved.

ISBN-13: 978-1546995142

ISBN-10: 1546995145

Contents

Disclaimer

We hope you enjoy reading our book, however we do suggest you read our disclaimer. All the material written in this book is provided for informational purposes only and is general in nature.

Every person is a unique individual and what has worked for some or even many may not work for you. Any information perceived as advice by must be considered in light of your own particular set of circumstances.

The author or person sharing this information does not assume any responsibility for the accuracy or outcome of your use of the content.

Every attempt has been made to provide well researched and up to date content at the time of writing. Now all the legalities have been taken care of, please enjoy the content.

See your healthcare professional before starting any diet, health or exercise program!

Introduction

There has never been a time in history when so many people have had so much *potential* control over their rate of aging as now. Knowledge is power – and the knowledge is available to those who want it.

Our bodies do not age or degenerate at the same rate, nor do they age in a linear progression. Our lives may be measured in years, but two people of the same chronological age may manifest very different biomarkers – the measurable statistics that reveal our physical age, rather than our chronological age.

While there are different factors that contribute to the rate our bodies age, such as environment (physical and mental/emotional), the biggest factor is proving to be diet. It is also the one we have the greatest control over, and can take action on the fastest.

Although this opportunity to extend our longevity exists, many people, even most, do not actively choose to exercise it. They will wish for it of course, but choosing to do it requires making mindful choices and taking action in regards to diet.

A big part of this action involves refraining from bad or poor choices as much as it does choosing good ones, and this can be the hardest part for most people.

This document outlines many of the foods proven to promote health and longevity.

The degree that any person can incorporate these super-foods into their diet, while at the same relinquishing damaging food types, will play a huge role in determining both length and quality of life.

Antioxidant Foods for A Youthful Appearance

Most people have the desire to maintain a youthful appearance as the years pass by. However, there are factors that usually make our youthful appearance disappear or diminish as we age.

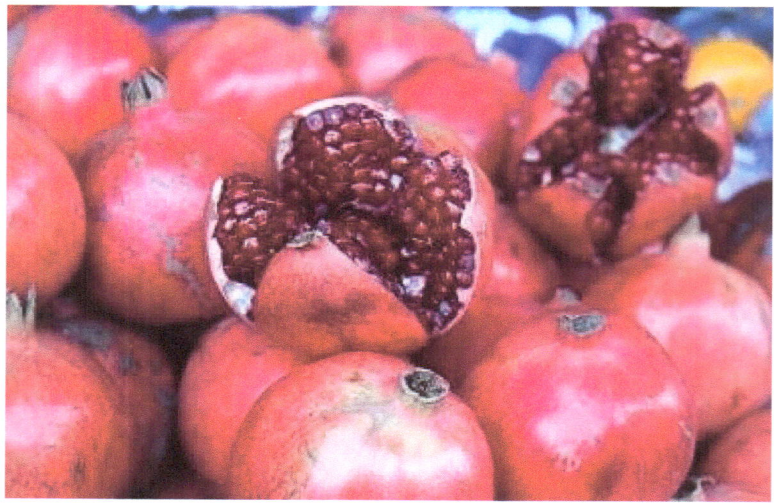

Damage to our skin from free radicals, losing and regaining weight, the sun's harmful rays and an unhealthy diet can take its toll on the whole body, and especially its protective outer coating the skin.

Antioxidants, known as phytochemicals, help protect the skin from sun damage and also helps repair the skin if sun damage occurs.

Therefore, one of the best ways to maintain a youthful appearance as you progress into old age is to choose foods high in antioxidants. Eating the right foods is the best way to guard against aging skin, wrinkles and age spots.

Add These Antioxidant Foods To Your Diet Plan

Here are some foods you can include in your anti-aging diet:

Pomegranates – The high levels of vitamin C in pomegranates make them an excellent source for fighting wrinkles. They contain punicalagin and ellagic acid which keeps the body's collagen healthy – which, in turn, helps your skin appear smooth and wrinkle-free.

Red Bell Peppers – These brightly colored vegetables are the perfect source for treating your skin to its daily requirement of vitamin C. Vitamin C helps your body absorb moisture which prevents dryness and subsequent wrinkles.

Fish – Cold water fish are especially helpful for reducing redness caused by skin inflammations such as psoriasis and eczema. Oily fish, such as mackerel and salmon, also contain omega 3 fatty acids to keep moisture in the skin-cells which helps strengthen them.

Avocados – Eating only one avocado every week can help your skin remain hydrated, soft and smooth by serving to maintain the cell membranes of the skin. One a day is even better!

Kale and Spinach – Look no further than kale and spinach for the phytonutrients and anti-oxidative compounds you need to prevent sun damage and maintain skin firmness. Increase skin elasticity with servings of spinach, which contains beta-carotene and lutein.

Blueberries – These little blue berries are powerhouses of antioxidants which are needed to provide extra protection from free radicals. Free radicals damage the skin and cause fine lines and wrinkles. Antioxidants can even help protect you from the ravages that emotional stress or over-exercising can cause to the body.

Green Tea – Drink plenty of green tea to help diminish brown spots, otherwise known as age spots. It's a healthy brew which contains effective ingredients for preventing sun and free radical damage.

Olive Oil – The good fats present in olive oil can keep that youthful glow on your face and provide you with omega 3 fatty acids to improve circulation beneath the skin. Use olive oil in salad dressings and when cooking to keep your skin rosy and healthy.

The truth is that you can spend all the money you have on potions, lotions, creams and masks, but only if you address the problems from the inside out – with a good healthy diet plan – can you truly hope to keep a youthful appearance.

If you want to remain looking young and healthy, create your own anti-aging diet plan. Add all the foods you need to, such as those mentioned above, and remove the ones that you know are not going to do you any good at all.

Beta Carotene – Anti-Aging Benefits and Foods

Experts agree that the main cause of aging and its visible effects is free radicals causing oxidative stress on the body. Look no further than the carotenoid, beta carotene, to stave off the damaging effects of free radicals on your entire body.

What Is Beta Carotene?

Beta carotene is considered a pro-vitamin – which simply means that it is not a vitamin in its present form, but can be converted to a vitamin by an organism. Beta carotene is water soluble and is converted to vitamin A in your body.

Its powerful anti-aging properties work with other antioxidants such as lipoic acid, vitamin E and C and antioxidant enzymes which are produced by the body. While many antioxidants provide some benefit in isolation, almost all are strongly boosted in efficiency by the presence of others.

The more complete the diet, the more complete the anti-aging protection.

Beta Carotene Anti-aging Health Benefits

The health benefits of beta carotene can prevent premature aging by:

- Providing relief from stress-related injuries (including carpal tunnel)

- Protect against damaging UV radiation from the sun

- Help prevent osteoarthritis, cataracts, diabetes and macular degeneration.

Scientific studies also show that beta carotene can help:

- The immune system to function properly

- Prevent some types of cancer

- Improve functions of the prostate

- Reduce pain and inflammation

- Increase your strength and endurance levels.

Beta Carotene Food Sources

You can find great dietary sources of beta carotene in some readily available and inexpensive foods such as dark green leafy vegetables, carrots, squash, cabbage and sweet potatoes. The antioxidant properties of these foods are very helpful in preventing premature aging of the skin.

Cooking the vegetables releases the carotene from the vegetables' fiber content and supplies more beta carotene to the body. It is always best to get your beta carotene with natural whole foods.

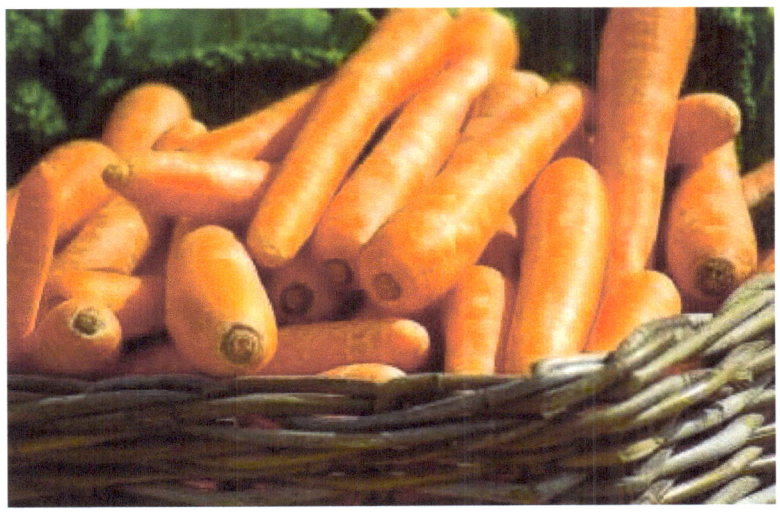

However, if you suspect you're not consuming enough of these super anti-aging foods, you may like to consider some of the green superfood powder supplements. These consist of wheat grass, chlorella, spirulina and barley. You can blend it into a super healthy smoothie by mixing it with fruit and perhaps some protein powder.

Additional Benefits

Besides helping cell-renewal of the skin, beta carotene also helps your pores stay unclogged, fade aging spots and scars and helps you maintain a glowing, healthy look to the skin.

Doctors are now prescribing diets high in beta carotene for certain maladies such as asthma, bronchitis and emphysema, male and female infertility, AIDS, cervical and prostate cancer and more.

As more research into the amazing benefits of beta carotene is conducted, more anti-aging benefits are sure to be revealed. Beta carotene is certainly a hot topic among those interested in slowing down the aging process, and you are bound to hear more about its anti-aging powers in the future.

So get started right now and be sure to include beta carotene rich foods into your anti-aging daily diet plan. There's no time like the present to make the clock stand still!

Boron Rich Foods for Anti-Aging

You may be unfamiliar with boron and its importance in keeping you young in appearance and body. Boron is a trace mineral which is used by several areas of the body including skin, bone and muscle.

Although boron isn't as well-known as its macro counterparts (magnesium and calcium), it plays a definite role in keeping you stay young and healthy. Ongoing research is cementing the knowledge that without essential trace elements such as boron, the body cannot properly utilize the macro nutrients.

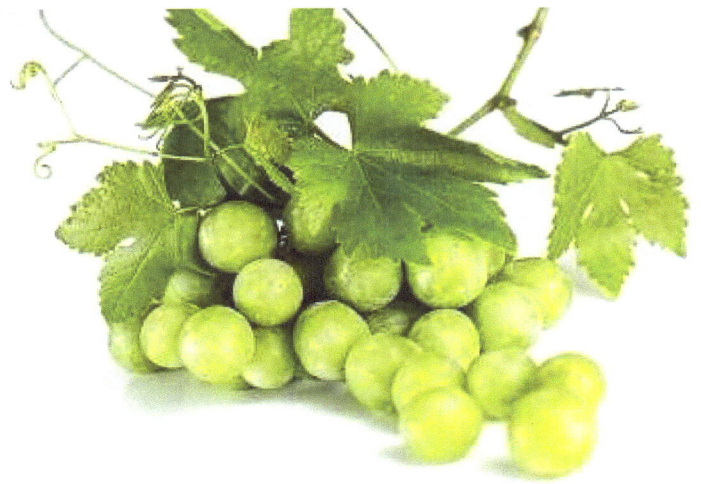

This means that in the absence of these essential micro-nutrients, increased intake of calcium will be excreted, and provide little benefit in bone building or other functions. As maintaining a strong skeleton is essential to delaying the effects of aging, it is important to look beyond mega-doses of calcium as the sole solution for overcoming osteoporosis.

Health Benefits of Boron

Some health and anti-aging benefits of boron include:

Protects Bones and Joints – Only 3 milligrams of boron per day helps to reduce the amount of calcium and magnesium that are lost in urinary excretion, indicating that it can help reduce the risk of bone deterioration during menopausal years. It also increases hormone serum levels and testosterone levels.

Balances Hormonal Levels – Both sexes can benefit from boron's power to level sex hormones. For women, boron helps to relieve menopausal symptoms and PMS.

Concentration and Brain Function – Aging adults may benefit from boron by its ability to help with attention span, retaining information, cognitive issues and revitalizing a sluggish brain. Research has proven that task performances, including motor skills, dexterity and perception can all be increased with boron.

Muscle Mass Improvement – Healthy muscle mass is important – especially as you age. With boron, vitamins and minerals are more readily absorbed and used by the body. You'll also have less pain following intense workouts, and it promotes testosterone production and higher energy levels.

Prevention and Treatment of Yeast Infections – Yeast infections have long been a problem for women. Boric acid is the form of boron used to heal infections in the vagina and is safe and effective.

Treats Diabetes – Changes in blood glucose and triglyceride levels may all be helped by increasing boron levels. It's also being tested for treatment of insulin resistance in some sufferers of diabetes.

Heals Skin – Skin irritation may be effectively treated with boron and it can even be used as an eye wash for infections or damaging bacteria. Boron may help to relieve skin irritation, redness and inflammation.

Digestive Disorders – Boron can rid your digestive tract of parasites which cause digestive distress such as upset stomach and other disorders.

Boron Rich Foods to Add To Your Diet

Boron is a natural substance found in whole foods such as whole grains, avocados, beans, berries, nuts, plums, grapes and oranges.

It's sometimes found in water in certain regions, but most of our boron comes to us through eating the right foods in our diet.

The boron we derive from the plants we eat is mainly boric acid.

More research is now being conducted to discover other benefits of boron on the human body, but we do know that it's ability to reduce signs of aging is undisputed.

Can Red Wine Keep You Young?

We've all heard at some point in time that red wine contains some sort of miracle ingredient that will help us to stay young. So all we need to do is to drink a glass of red wine every day and enjoy the anti-aging benefits. However, is this right or wrong?

Well, the verdict is still out with some scientific researchers on whether red wine can help us maintain our youth. There's no doubt, however, that a glass of red wine per day for women and one or two for men provides some of the anti-aging properties which intervene with the aging process.

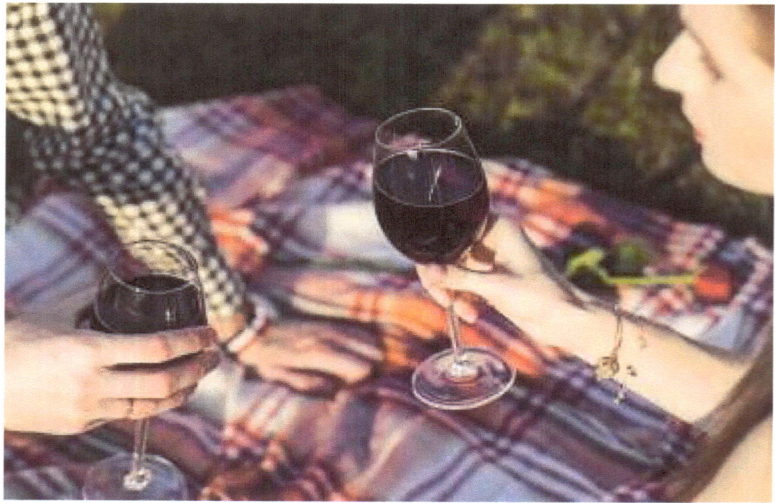

The healthiest people on earth – those who live in the Mediterranean region – enjoy a lifestyle which includes a glass of red wine along with fresh fruits, vegetables and fish. They also tend to have less stress in their lives, which can also play a huge part in keeping the aging process at bay.

As you can see, it's not all about the wine!

Antioxidants In Red Wine - Resveratrol

Antioxidant foods are known to be helpful, even essential, in age prevention. They help soak up the free radicals which are some of the major causes of aging and age-related diseases. Red wine contains a higher concentration of polyphenols and resveratrol (antioxidants) than plain grape juice.

The reason red wine is better than plain old grape juice is because of the way wine is produced. The skin and seeds are removed when making grape juice – but left as part of the fermenting process when making wine.

A Glass of Red Wine and The Benefits

The benefits of drinking the recommended amount of red wine per day doesn't stop at just giving you a 'healthy' glow. Statistics show that you may live an average of five years longer than a person who doesn't imbibe.

You'll also statistically have fewer pre-cancerous skin lesions and expect a lower risk of cancer, diabetes and Alzheimer's disease or dementia. It actually shows that those who drink red wine on a regular basis have an 80% lower chance of developing dementia-related diseases during old age.

If You Don't Like Red Wine, What Can You Do?

If for any reason you can't drink red wine, you can still choose to add the types of foods to your diet which have lots of polyphenols and antioxidants -- like blueberries or dark chocolate.

There are also resveratrol supplements, but not enough research has been done on whether they have the same effect as drinking red wine.

If you're a white wine drinker, you should know that white wines have less antioxidant properties than the reds. Also, if you're thinking of switching to red wine for the health benefits, the higher levels of polyphenols are more prevalent in European wines than American.

Red wine is also known to help the digestive process – which may be another reason the Mediterranean population is so healthy as they enjoy a glass of red wine with every meal.

Don't Over-Indulge

However, beware of too much of a good thing. While drinking a glass of red wine once per day may provide you with antioxidants, drinking too much wine can undo all the good you might receive and have a detrimental effect on your health and anti-aging efforts.

You certainly don't want to gain excess weight from over-indulging, as this causes other health problems. Plus, you don't want it to become an addiction where you look forward to that night-cap.

Add Dates to Your Anti-aging Diet

For centuries, dates have been eaten to benefit sexual drive, promote weight gain and to build muscles. They're also delicious to eat by themselves or to spiff up a bowl of oatmeal or other dishes. However, the health benefits of dates are monumental.

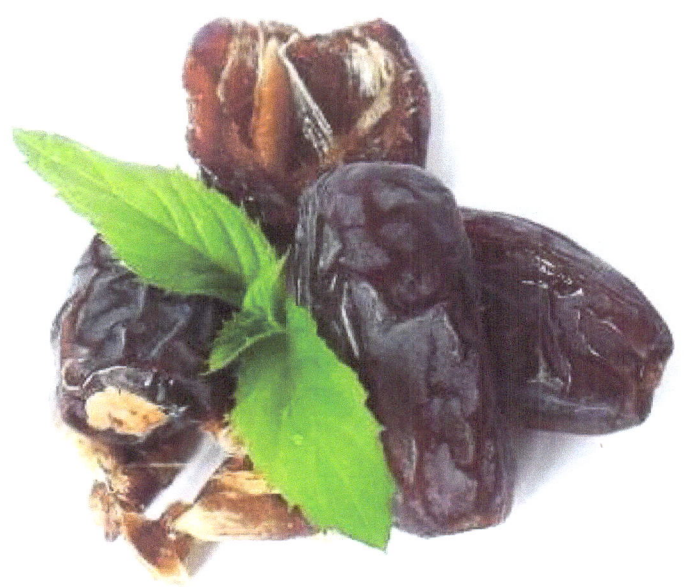

Dates are the fruits of various varieties of palm trees, and are highly-prized in Middle Eastern and North African cultures and folklore. The palm varieties that provide the dates most consumers are familiar with traditionally grow in desert regions. Palm trees from tropical regions produce different but related fruits, such as acai berries.

The Health Benefits of Adding Dates to Your Anti-aging Diet

Some ways that eating dates can improve your health and help you stay young include:

Healthy Heart – Cholesterol clogs the arteries and puts you at risk for heart disease. Dates contain potassium which reduces risk of stroke and lowers bad LDL cholesterol levels.

Bones and Blood – Lower your risk of cancer and keep your bones young and strong by eating dates. They contain manganese, selenium and magnesium – dates are a super food for anti-aging.

Digestive Health – Keep your digestive system humming with the soluble fiber in dates. This fiber keeps water in the digestive system and is great for alleviating constipation and maintaining bowel regularity. Potassium rich dates also help relieve diarrhea and upset stomachs. Dates also help create good bacteria in the stomach to help maintain optimal gut flora.

Boost Your Energy Level – Natural sugars in dates make them the perfect snack to perk up your energy levels when you're feeling fatigued. Fiber in dates keep your energy levels up without suffering from the usual crash you might experience with other sugary, unhealthy snacks.

Boost Iron Level – Anemia is a condition that results from low iron levels and can leave you feeling run down and constantly fatigued. Dates are a great source of iron and are an excellent source for helping to boost your iron and energy levels.

Relieve Allergies – Seasonal allergies can put you out of commission for days or even weeks at a time. Dates have been proven to help relieve the annoying symptoms of allergies and improve your fight against them.

Alleviate Sexual Dysfunction – Skeptics question the aphrodisiac powers of dates, but research indicates that the estradiol and flavonoid compounds found in dates may increase sexual function. Definitely worth a try, don't you think?

Natural Antioxidants and Antibacterial Properties – The antioxidant and antibacterial power of dates are crucial to keeping your body and skin young and free from bacteria-related illnesses.

As you can see, reaching for a snack of dates can be far more beneficial to your health and age prevention than eating a processed snack bar. Dates are also an excellent source of vitamins and minerals essential for maintaining good health.

When you add dates to your diet, you are enriching your diet with all sorts of minerals such as magnesium, calcium, iron, phosphorus, zinc and potassium – all of which are necessary to keep you healthy as you age.

Eat Nuts to Help Keep a Youthful Appearance

Nuts are delicious, and it's nice to know you can eat nuts to help keep a youthful appearance! Your diet directly affects your appearance and – if you choose correctly – your diet can help you remain youthful as you age.

Nuts are often avoided because of the fear they contain too much fat, but the reality is that some nuts have incredible anti-aging properties and you only have to eat a few each day to get the results. There is also increasing evidence that the fat in nuts is beneficial to health and longevity.

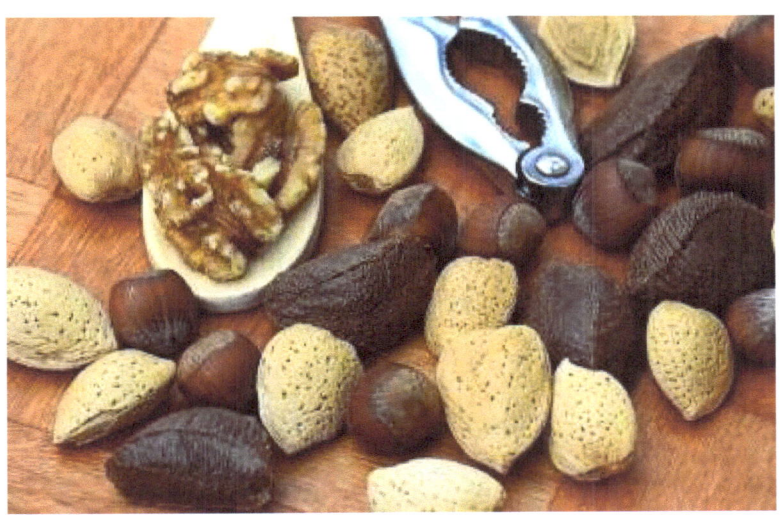

Brazil Nuts, Walnuts and More

Brazil nuts contain selenium which helps heal wounds and boost your skin and overall health. They can also help the thyroid glands keep active and function properly, and if you eat a couple of ounces of shelled walnuts every day, your blood vessels will remain more flexible and healthy.

Nuts contain benefits such as keeping you healthier, improving your sex life, kidneys, brain power, heart and also helps you keep that youthful glow.

Consuming about 2.5 ounces of nuts on a daily basis helps to lower your cholesterol, boost the ratio of HDL heart-friendly lipoproteins, lowers damaging low-density lipoproteins and even helps to lower your triglyceride levels.

Here are some other great effects that nuts can have on your body and overall health:

Pistachios – Consuming about 2 or 3 ounces of pistachios per day helps to lower LDL (bad) and raise HDL (good) cholesterol levels.

Hazelnuts – Lower your risk of heart disease by munching on a handful of hazelnuts each day and also protect yourself from some forms of dementia and cancers.

Almonds – Helps preserve the good HDL cholesterol levels and lower the bad LDL cholesterol levels.

One of the healthiest population centers in the world is that found in the Mediterranean region. This is one of the reasons why there are many advocates that follow a 'Mediterranean Diet'.

Along with the other healthy diet choices that Mediterranean locals eat, this population consumes an average of 30 grams of nuts per day.

Why Do Some People Fear Eating Nuts?

Some people avoid eating nuts because of their fear of weight gain, but nuts actually have very little effect on weight gain. Nuts have sometimes received a bad rap because they are known to be high in fat – but nuts contain fats that shouldn't be regarded as unhealthy.

Nuts are also great sources of protein and fiber and are proven to provide many health benefits, including the ones we have mentioned in regards to lowering the risk of heart disease.

Great Mineral and Vitamin Source

Other vitamins and minerals contained in nuts include magnesium and vitamin E – great resources to keep your skin young and glowing. Health-wise, nuts are known to lower the risk of some metabolic conditions such as high cholesterol and high blood pressure.

Therefore, include more nuts in your anti-aging diet. They're satisfying and delicious and can help prevent many chronic diseases. It is always a bonus to eat a snack that tastes great, and is good for you too!

Omega 3 Anti-Aging Benefits and Foods

The body doesn't have the ability to manufacture essential omega 3 fatty acids (also known as polyunsaturated fatty acids – PUFA), so they must be obtained from the foods you eat.

Omega 3 fatty acids are necessary for the body to carry out its proper functions and are also crucial for brain function.

Our body's cells become thin and less able to stick together as we age, causing our skin to become dry and saggy. Omega 3 fatty acids help the body's outer layer (epidermis) to retain moisture and to repair itself when needed.

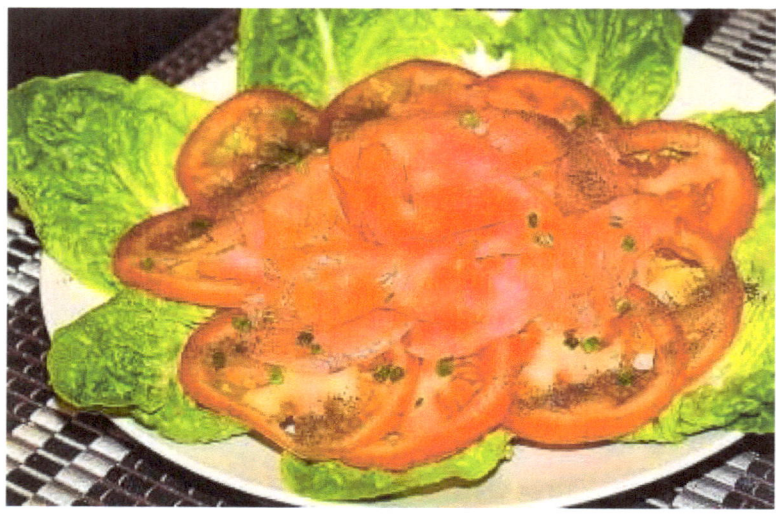

More Health Benefits

Besides the benefits to the skin, omega 3 helps reduce the risk of heart disease and other diseases such as arthritis, diabetes and cancer.

These powerful omega 3 fatty acids also reduce inflammation in the body and prevent sun damage to the skin.

Omega 3 Rich Foods

Omega 3 fatty acids can be found in salmon, sardines and a few plant foods such as seeds and nuts. High-quality beef also contains a fair amount of omega 3.

As consumers have begun to realize the importance of omega 3 fatty acids in their diets, food producers are touting the benefits of the omega 3 content in their products.

You'll find that omega 3 may be artificially added to some processed foods such as cereal, peanut butter, baby formula and others.

Keep in mind that it's best to get your vitamins – including omega 3 -- from natural sources of food, including seafood. But, while it isn't as ideal, you can choose some foods fortified with omega 3 to be sure you're getting your daily intake.

Some fruit juices, eggs, yogurt, weight loss drinks and pasteurized dairy products are fortified with this essential vitamin. Also, some omega 3s are now being added to animal feed so you'll get even higher levels in your dairy, poultry and meat products.

If your diet, fortified or otherwise, is lacking in this all-important nutrient, you can take supplements to be sure you're getting the recommended 4,000 milligrams per day.

Studies show that some of the healthiest populations on earth live in areas where foods containing omega 3 fatty acids are abundant.

The Mediterranean population (Spain, Greece, Turkey, France and Italy) is considered to be one of the healthiest and happiest populations on earth – there are many dietary reasons, but one more is because of the omega 3 rich foods they consume.

If You Don't Get Enough

If you are not getting enough omega 3 fatty acids in your diet it means you run the risk of contracting many of the maladies which affect us in our elder years including high blood pressure, buildup of cholesterol in the blood vessels, bone and joint pain, lack of concentration and learning ability and a less than adequate immune system.

Feel better, improve your appearance and keep aging at bay by taking steps to include adequate omega 3 in your diet plan.

Vitamin C - Anti-Aging Benefits and Foods

Vitamin C is one of the antioxidant vitamins that neutralize the free radicals which damage the cells of the body and skin.

Although many cosmetic creams and lotions claim to contain Vitamin C, the content tends to be very low and the final result isn't much help at all. Scientists have found that applying antioxidant-rich vitamins to your skin in the form of creams or lotions aren't very well absorbed and that the beneficial effects are short-lived.

To get the full anti-aging advantage of vitamin C, you should consume it, rather than apply it. Therefore, choose foods that contain vitamin C and benefit from both the inside to the outside!

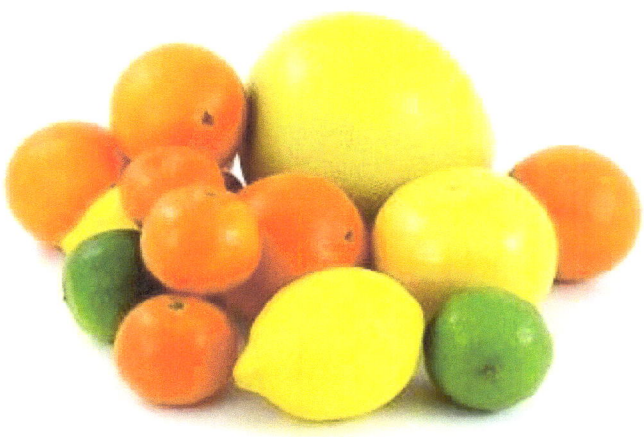

Vitamin C Foods to Add To Your Diet

Some of the best vitamin C-rich foods to add to your anti-aging diet include citrus fruits and vegetables.

Foods such as dark leafy greens, all citrus fruits, tomatoes, bell peppers, berries and kiwifruit contain high amounts of vitamin C.

The Anti-Aging Benefits

These foods contribute to the creation of ATP, peptide hormones, dopamine and tyrosine – all highly effective in cell restoration and oxidation purposes.

With vitamin C, you'll get the added benefits of lowering your risk of cancer, reducing scar tissue and helping to maintain cartilage and blood vessels.

As a powerful anti-oxidant, vitamin C fights the molecules known as free radicals to keep their activity from becoming excessive and damaging cells and tissue.

Other examples of damage that can be caused by free radicals include our DNA (genetic matter) and damage to the eyes' lenses – all which could possibly be prevented by the adequate consumption of vitamin C.

Vitamin C has also been proven to increase the absorption of iron in the intestine. Being able to absorb iron properly can also help reduce the effects of aging.

What Happens If You Don't Get Enough Vitamin C?

Despite most people understanding the importance of vitamin C, and that it can be found readily available in citrus fruits, many people still don't get enough in their daily diet to fully benefit from its powerful healing properties.

This lack of vitamin C can cause health problems, from minor to severe, depending on the degree of deficiency.

Collagen, which is the critical protein that frames our skin and bones, requires vitamin C to produce it. Therefore, a deficiency will cause skin problems and increased visible signs of aging.

Extreme vitamin C deficiencies leads to conditions such as scurvy. Those with scurvy begin to lose teeth, lose their muscle strength, tend to bleed easily and suffer other life-threatening problems. Fortunately, a small amount of vitamin C (even just one lime per day) is enough to prevent this.

Vitamin C is also necessary for complete brain health, another important body component to keep healthy as you age! It helps produce neurotransmitters in the brain which transmit signals of our feelings and thoughts to the body's nervous system.

It also produces serotonin, the hormone that helps our immune system, endocrine and digestive systems.

It's vitally important to your health and longevity that you include vitamin C-rich foods in your diet on a daily basis as part of your anti-aging and overall well-being plan.

If for any reason your diet is deficient in these foods, supplementation is recommended to ensure adequate intake of this essential nutrient.

What Are the Best Anti-aging Foods?

You can add quality years to your life by changing your diet to include some of nature's most age-reducing, life-supporting foods. They will help to keep you energized and provide the nutrients you need to slow down the aging process and prevent diseases that normally affect the aged, such as arthritis and heart disease.

Begin by adding some of the healthiest foods on the planet to your daily food choices. Antioxidant abundant foods such as olive oil, berries, nuts and yogurt are delicious and very easy to incorporate into any diet either in meals or as a nutritious snack.

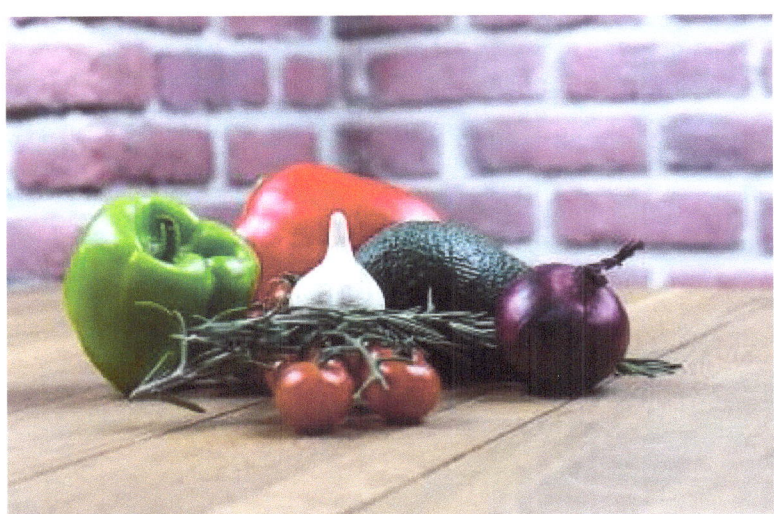

Add These Delicious, Nutritious Anti-Aging Foods to Your Diet

Some great anti-aging food choices and what they can do for you include:

Berries – Rich in antioxidants and able to fight the free radicals that can ruin your immune system; berries are one of your best defenses against the aging process.

Garlic – An herb with an attitude, garlic has an impressive list of anti-aging properties. Healing is one of its best attributes – and it can help to prevent colds and boost your immune system.

Red Wine – Drinking red wine in moderation is a health benefit with anti-aging properties which include resveratrol, shown to slow cellular aging by activating certain genes.

Yogurt – Make sure it's all natural acidophilus yogurt, not the sweetened varieties. The acidophilus yogurt is helpful in providing the calcium component of your diet, which may help prevent osteoporosis. It also contains the good bacteria to help you maintain digestive health and reduce the risk of intestinal diseases.

Fish – Good for the heart, fish (especially salmon and other oily fish) contains omega 3 fatty acids, which help prevent the buildup of cholesterol in the arteries. Fish also contain antioxidants which are known to help fight the aging process.

Nuts – Increasing brain function is vital to slowing the aging process. Nuts contain omega 3 fatty acids which help to increase brain function and also have a high concentration of minerals, antioxidants, vitamins and phytochemicals which further delay signs of aging.

Legumes – Fiber-rich beans have been proven to lower cholesterol and provide good bacteria to your body. Legumes are inexpensive and very satisfying as a meal.

Dark Chocolate – Contains flavanols that serve to help the blood vessels function as they should. When you take care of the blood vessels, you'll stave off the risk of high blood pressure, dementia, kidney disease and type 2 diabetes. Just remember to eat in moderation! Although it's on the good list, you'll risk weight gain if you over indulge.

Leafy Green Vegetables – These high-fiber vegetables are rich in nutrients which can serve to halt the aging process. Choose from kale, spinach, cabbage, broccoli and turnip greens to spiff up your diet with anti-aging helpers.

Taking steps to exercise anti-aging diet measures that will slow the aging process isn't difficult. Choosing from the above foods and adding them to your daily diet plan is the best way to keep your body and mind healthy. That way you can progress through your senior years empowered and strong.

Which Foods Fight Wrinkles?

Believe it or not, you might enjoy fighting wrinkles by making a few dietary changes. You can choose to eat some delicious key foods which delay the aging process and improve your skin condition. Good skin must have a sufficient supply of the right nutrients to successfully fight the telltale signs of aging – wrinkles.

Spending a fortune on topical solutions will never be enough. You've heard it all before, 'you are what you eat' and that includes eating bad foods that can cause prematurely aging skin.

Adding certain foods to your diet works better than any cream or procedure and of course makes you healthier all over.

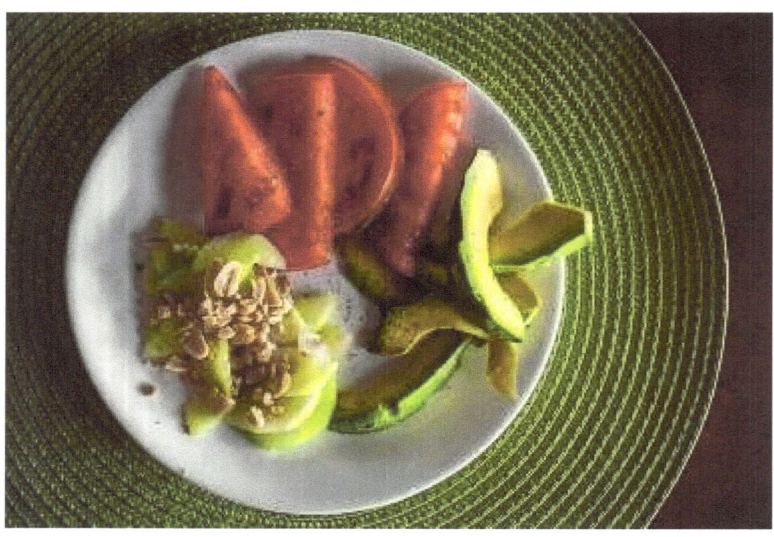

Add These Wrinkle Fighting Foods to Your Diet

Some foods that fight aging and help to revitalize your skin and prevent wrinkles include:

Tomatoes – Vitamin C and lycopene are the keys to a tomatoes success in keeping your skin firm and plump. Vitamin C helps to build collagen and lycopene prevents UV damage and boosts the vascular system.

Avocados – These are one of those foods that are packed with incredible goodies for your skin and health. High in glutathione, avocados are great for detoxing the body and flushing harmful toxins from your system. Glutathione may also help acne as well as prevent wrinkles – plus, help prevent some cancers.

Green Tea – Drink green tea for its detoxifying properties and the age-defying chemical called EGCG. Green tea can regenerate your cells, help them grow and stay healthy during their lives. If not cared for properly, your body's cells can deteriorate and increase your risk for cancer and skin pigmentation.

Honey – Taken internally as a sweetener rather than sugar, honey acts as an antioxidant and anti-viral boost to your system. Sugar causes inflammation, but honey is good for you. You can also use honey as a face mask to clear impurities from your pores and plump fine lines and wrinkles.

Berries – Packed with flavonoids, antioxidants, vitamins, probiotics and polyphenols, berries are known as "free radical scavengers." Toxins in your environment can wreak havoc on your skin. Berries help the skin to regenerate and stave off wrinkles.

Rooibos Tea – Premature aging may be prevented or slowed by drinking rooibos tea to hydrate the skin and protect it from free radicals. Many people drink it as a substitute for coffee, which is very dehydrating.

Kefir – Fights irritations and redness of the skin with its friendly bacteria and probiotics. Kefir is similar to yogurt, but contains more probiotics. Be sure to choose unprocessed and natural foods (including kefir and yogurt) to enjoy the highest levels of probiotics.

Remove Sugary, High-Processed Foods From Your Diet

Excess sugar in your diet will help cause wrinkles and hasten the aging process.

Remove high-processed foods from your diet too. They're not good for you, for too many reasons to list here, however, they do speed up the aging process and reduce your longevity.

It's important that you choose foods that will keep your skin hydrated – both inside and out and include those foods with omega 3, 6 and 9 fatty acids.

Aging gracefully (and slowly) depends greatly on the foods you choose. Choose wisely and you'll keep the youthful, dewy complexion you desire. People will be letting you know just how great you look for your age!

Final Thoughts

Growing older in years is not a choice, we are all going there. However, it is exciting to realize that we have a large degree of control over not only how long we can live, but how vital we can be while we are alive.

Vitality lets us enjoy our life – living rather than simply existing. What we eat can play a massive part in this. Poor food choices are making many people's lives a struggle every day, as they deal with the effects of so-called lifestyle diseases.

By letting go of the foods that we know are injurious to our health, and replacing them more and more with the foods discussed above, we can age more productively, with stronger bodies and sharper minds.

Other Relevant Books by This Author

If you would like to read more relevant books about this topic, here is a list of the Amazon paperback links, titles and descriptions from this author:

https://www.createspace.com/6986819

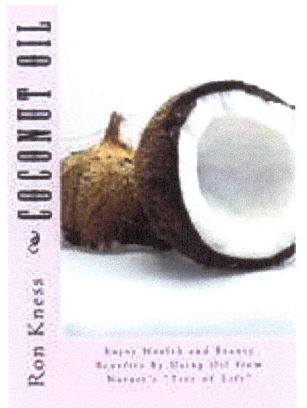

Coconut Oil: Enjoy Health and Beauty Benefits By Using Oil from Nature's "Tree of Life"

We want to be thankful for nature's bounty of the versatile oil. We also want to be more in control of our health and looks.

And we want to enjoy all the benefits coconut oil provides! We can achieve ALL of these goals with the newest release from Ron Kness called "Coconut Oil - Enjoy Health Benefits And More From Nature's Tree Of Life".

Based on these exciting teachings, you will learn about all the dramatic benefits of health from using coconut oil as part of a healthy eating plan and looking good from using coconut oil as an integral part of a beauty and anti-aging regimen.

This book is built around a very clear, concept: enjoy life to its fullest by using coconut oil to not only feel good, but also look good. It's not just about the benefits of using this often misunderstood natural-occurring oil.

Having great looks and health as you age is linked to being happy and full of life. This is because using coconut oil helps heal the body both inside and out In this book, we look at all of the ways you can improve your own looks and health as you age, starting with knowing how and when to use coconut oil.

This book also looks at the many other steps that can be taken to support this goal, from selecting the right type of coconut oil for the purpose intended, to continuing to use other holistic methods of beauty and healing as part of a healthy lifestyle, such as essential oils and aromatherapy.

The choices you make about using coconut oil today will have a significant impact on your looks and health as you age. In "Coconut Oil - Enjoy Health Benefits And More From Nature's Tree Of Life", we'll cover all the bases, giving you everything you need to know to use coconut oil to improve both your looks, health, and ultimately your life!

https://www.createspace.com/6345319

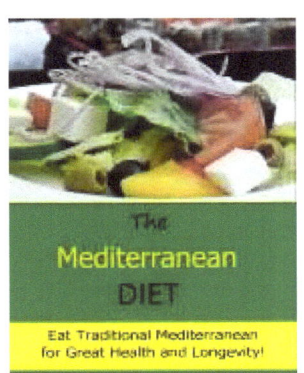

The Mediterranean Diet: Eat Traditional Mediterranean for Great Health and Longevity!

The Mediterranean Diet is one of the very best diets there is for anyone who wants to lose weight in a way that's healthy, fun and sustainable.

This is a diet that's all about treating food with respect and all about getting natural ingredients in a way that you can actually enjoy. And the benefits of that are incredible. The numbers speak for themselves but it goes beyond just lifespan and heart health. This is a diet that can make you feel the best you've felt in years. Somewhere along the way, our approach to diet here in the US has become twisted.

I'm talking about our general diet sure but I'm also talking about our attempts to eat healthily and lose weight! And in many ways, our diet is a reflection of our lifestyle: everything is fast, convenient and consumable. At the same time though, it lacks substance and it lacks passion. We have lost respect for our diet and we've stopped seeing food as something to be enjoyed.

Instead, we see it as an inconvenience. We're too busy to eat – and so we grab the quickest thing to eat from the cupboard or the fridge. Normally that means eating ready-made meals that are full of sugar and processed meats, or it means eating Mars Bars that literally offer us zero nutrition. Unsurprisingly, this leads to many of us gaining a lot of weight as all we're eating is sugar and in high quantities.

At the same time, our skin, hair and nails look damaged because we aren't getting the bioavailable amino acids or the vitamins and minerals that we need. All that sugar has led to an epidemic of diabetes and many other preventable diseases are running rife.

Those of us who want to do something about this weight gain try to do so by counting calories or cutting fat. Now we're getting even less sustenance from our food while still feeling exhausted and burned out all the time. Now we feel guilty whenever we eat.

Now our relationship with our food is even worse. Scientists were very surprised when they looked at data from around the world and found that people who ate a Mediterranean Diet lived longer, were less likely to get heart disease and were thinner. But when you think about it, it's obvious! These are people who spend actual time cooking fresh, healthy meals. Many of those meals are PACKED with fruits, with vegetables, with salad and with fish.

These are all foods that are stuffed with nutrients. Nutrients that the body uses to build muscle, to regulate hormones, to provide energy and to improve our mood.

As soon as you start eating food that you enjoy – as soon as you slow down to smell the delicious garlic coming from your bolognaise – you begin eating well again and your body thanks you for it. Those living in the Mediterranean area have eaten this way for years and enjoy better health and more longevity than most in other areas ... there must be something to this way of living.

https://www.createspace.com/6867124

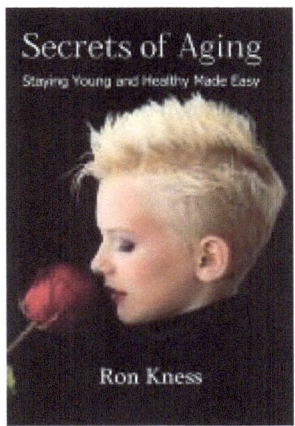

Secrets of Aging: Staying Young and Healthy Made Easy

We all want to be young and beautiful regardless of our age. We also want to be healthy. And we want to minimize the effects of aging!

We can achieve ALL of these goals with my newest book release "Secrets Of Aging". Based on these exciting teachings, you will learn about all the dramatic benefits of staying young looking by using a good skincare and beauty regimen and living a healthy lifestyle as a way of staying younger looking than your real age.

This book is built around a very clear, concept: look young and be healthy for as long as possible.

It's not just about methods used to reduce, and in some cases reverse, the effects of aging. Having great looks and health as we age is linked to living a healthy lifestyle and taking of ourselves .

This is possible with the use of proven anti-aging methods and products. In this book, we look at all of the ways you can improve your own looks and health as you age, starting with a healthy lifestyle. This book will also look at the many other steps that can be taken to support this goal, from eating healthy foods and using a skincare maintenance program, to dressing, using make-up and wearing a hairstyle appropriate for people your age.

The choices you make now about taking care of your body both inside and out has an impact on your looks and health as you age!

In "Secrets of Aging", we'll cover all the bases, giving you everything you need to know to use anti-aging tips and techniques to stay young and healthy for as long as possible.

About the Author

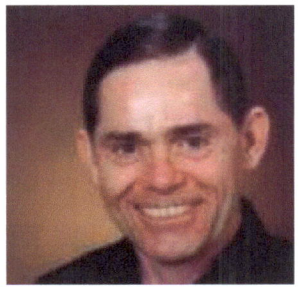

I have published over 125 books on Amazon for Kindle, CreateSpace and other publishing platforms.

While most of my books are on health and fitness in general, as I age (now 65) at the time of this writing) my topics of interest are geared toward aging baby boomers and older.

Besides my own writing, I also ghostwrite ebooks, books, reports, articles, blogs and do Kindle conversions for clients on a variety of topics.

Today my wife and I are retired from our careers and live in Gold Canyon, AZ. I now write as a retirement business where you'll find me happily sitting in my office typing away on my laptop as I work on my next book or ghostwriting project . . . that is if we are not traveling on a cruise ship - our new-found mode of travel.